21 MEDITERRANEAN DIET SHEET-PAN DINNERS TO HELP REDUCE INFLAMMATION

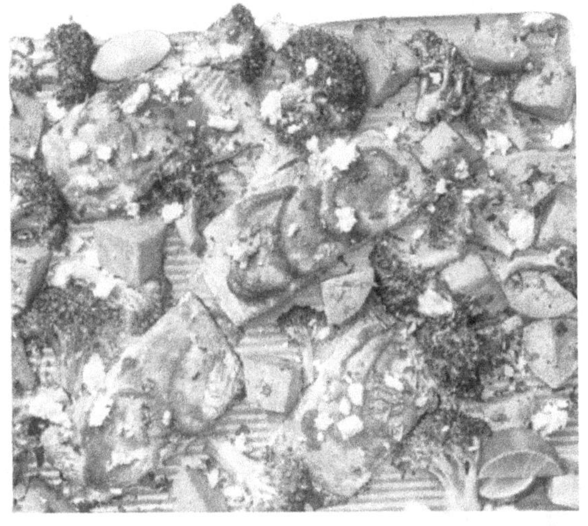

Dr. Malvin harison

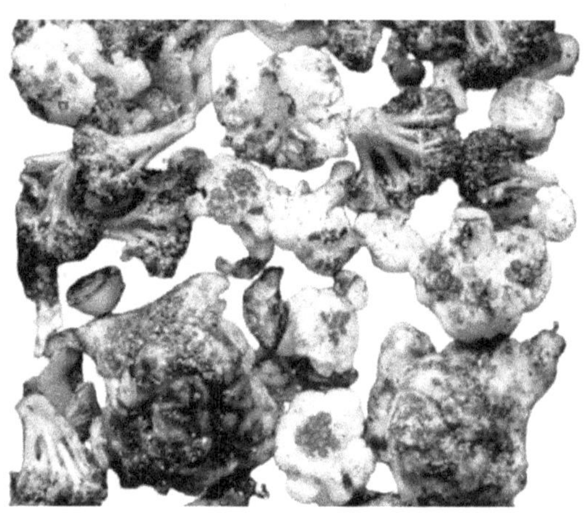

TABLE OF CONTENT

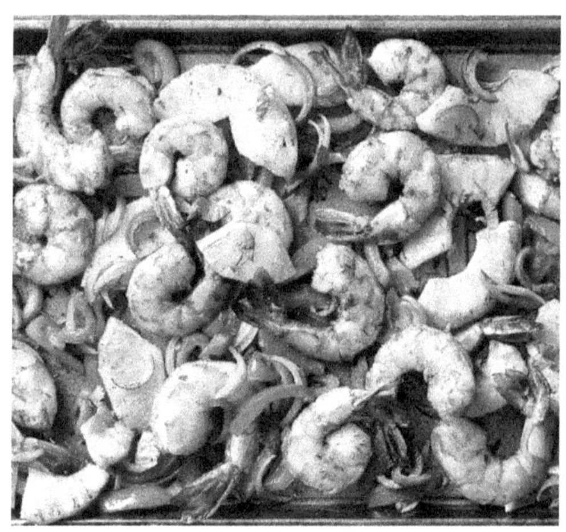

INTRODUCTION

These mitigating, Mediterranean eating regimen suppers can assist you with consolidating a wealth of sound fats, vegetables, flavors, vegetables, and entire grains in your eating design. Each dish is loaded with fixings like dull mixed greens, olive oil, and fish, which are perfect for combatting the side effects of persistent aggravation. Furthermore, these recipes are ready on a sheet skillet to help you all the more advantageously adjust your night feasts to one of the best eating designs on the planet. Recipes like our Zesty Jerk Shrimp and Garlic Broiled Salmon and Brussels Fledglings are nutritious and tasty supper choices you'll need to make over and over.

21 MEDITERRANEAN DIET SHEET-PAN DINNERS TO HELP REDUCE INFLAMMATION

1. Sheet pan Salmon with Yams and Broccoli

The lively combo of cheddar, cilantro, stew, and lime — roused by Mexican road corn — makes this salmon sheet-container supper burst with flavor.

Ingredients

3 tablespoons low-fat mayonnaise

1 teaspoon stew powder

2 medium yams, stripped and cut into 1-inch 3D squares

4 teaspoons olive oil, isolated

½ teaspoon salt, separated

¼ teaspoon ground pepper, separated

4 cups of broccoli florets (8 oz.; 1 medium crown)

1 ¼ pounds salmon filet, cut into 4 segments

2 limes, 1 zested and squeezed, 1 cut into wedges for serving

¼ cup disintegrated feta or cotija cheddar

½ cup cleaved new cilantro

Instructions

Preheat the stove to 425 degrees F. Line a large rimmed baking sheet with foil and coat with a cooking splash.

Join mayonnaise and bean stew powder in a little bowl. Put away.

Throw yams with 2 tsp. oil, 1/4 tsp. salt, and 1/8 tsp. pepper in a medium bowl.

Spread on the pre-arranged baking sheet. Broil for 15 minutes.

In the interim, throw broccoli with the excess 2 tsp. oil, 1/4 tsp. salt, and 1/8 tsp. pepper in a similar bowl.

Eliminate the baking sheet from the stove. Mix the yams and move them to the sides of the container. Orchestrate salmon in the focal point of the container and spread the broccoli on one or the other side, among the yams.

Spread 2 Tbsp. of the mayonnaise combination over the salmon.

Heat until the yams are delicate and the salmon chips effectively with a fork, around 15 minutes.

In the interim, add lime zing and lime juice to the leftover 1 Tbsp. mayonnaise; blend well.

Split the salmon between 4 plates and top with cheddar and cilantro.

Split the yams and broccoli between the plates and sprinkle with the lime-mayonnaise sauce. Present with lime wedges and any excess sauce.

2. Zesty Jerk Shrimp

This is a shrimp sheet container dinner that is broiled and caramelized flawlessly! The pineapple in this recipe makes a sweet sauce that adjusts the intensity of the Jamaican jerk preparation.

Ingredients

1 ½ pounds new or frozen enormous shrimp in shells

4 (1/4 inch thick) cuts stripped and cored new pineapple, divided

2 cups scaled-down strips of red sweet pepper

2 cups cut red onions

1 new jalapeño chile pepper, divided longwise, cultivated, and cut

2 tablespoons olive oil

1 tablespoon Jamaican jerk preparing

½ cup coarsely clipped new cilantro

1 ⅓ cups hot cooked earthy colored rice

Lime wedges

Instructions

Defrost shrimp, whenever frozen. Preheat the stove to 425 degrees F. Line two 15x10-inch baking containers with foil.

Strip and devein shrimp, leaving tails in one piece whenever wanted. Wash shrimp; wipe off. In an extra-huge bowl join shrimp and the following six fixings (through jerk preparing); throw tenderly to cover. Split the blend between the pre-arranged skillet. Cook for 15 minutes or until the shrimp are dark.

Sprinkle with cilantro and present with earthy-colored rice and lime wedges.

Tip: Chile peppers contain oils that can disturb your skin and eyes. Wear plastic or elastic gloves while working with them.

3.Sheet-pan balsamic-Parmesan Chicken and Vegetables

This tasty dish- - with the blend of balsamic vinegar and Parmesan cheddar - makes an incredible weeknight dinner since it requires little legwork (and just a single skillet!). The marjoram adds a particular hearty fragrance. On the off chance that you don't have marjoram in your zest armory, you can utilize dried oregano all things considered. Both taste really woodsy and praise the dish flawlessly.

Fixings

4 cups broccoli florets

3 cups cauliflower florets

1 cup cut shallots

3 tablespoons extra-virgin olive oil, isolated

½ teaspoon salt, isolated

½ teaspoon ground pepper, isolated

2 enormous cloves garlic, minced

1 teaspoon dried marjoram

4 enormous bone-in chicken thighs, skin eliminated whenever wanted

3 tablespoons balsamic vinegar

⅓ cup ground Parmesan cheddar

Instructions

Preheat the broiler to 450 degrees F. Cover an enormous rimmed baking sheet with a cooking shower.

Consolidate broccoli, cauliflower, shallots, 2 tablespoons oil, 1/4 teaspoon salt, and 1/4 teaspoon pepper in a huge bowl. Throw well to cover. Move to the pre-arranged baking sheet.

Join garlic, marjoram, and the leftover 1 tablespoon oil and 1/4 teaspoon each salt and pepper in a little bowl. Cover the two sides of the chicken with the garlic combination. Put on the baking sheet. Cook the chicken and vegetables for about 15 minutes. Throw the vegetables and sprinkle the chicken with vinegar. Sprinkle all with Parmesan and keep simmering until the vegetables are delicate and a moment-read thermometer embedded in the thickest piece of the chicken without contacting bone registers 165 degrees F, around 10 additional minutes.

4. Garlic Broiled Salmon and Brussels Fledglings

Broiling salmon on top of Brussels fledglings and garlic, enhanced with wine and new oregano, is straightforward enough for a weeknight dinner yet complex enough to organize. Present with entire wheat couscous.

Fixings

14 huge cloves of garlic, isolated

¼ cup extra-virgin olive oil

2 tablespoons finely cleaved new oregano, isolated

1 teaspoon salt, partitioned

¾ teaspoon newly ground pepper, partitioned

6 cups Brussels grows, managed, and cut

¾ cup white wine, ideally Chardonnay

2 pounds wild-caught salmon filet, cleaned, cut into 6 segments

Lemon wedges

Instructions

Preheat the stove to 450 degrees F.

Mince 2 garlic cloves and join in a little bowl with oil, 1 tablespoon oregano, 1/2 teaspoon salt, and 1/4 teaspoon pepper. Divide the leftover garlic and throw with Brussels fledglings and 3 tablespoons of the carefully prepared oil in an enormous cooking skillet. Broil, mixing once, for 15 minutes.

Add wine to the excess oil blend. Eliminate the skillet from the stove, mix the vegetables, and put salmon on top. Shower with the wine blend. Sprinkle with the leftover 1 tablespoon oregano and 1/2 teaspoon each salt and pepper. Prepare until the salmon is simply cooked through, 5 to 10 minutes more. Present with lemon wedges.

5. 15-Minute Sheet pan Chicken strips and Broccoli.

Supper is prepared in just 15 minutes and cleanup is a breeze with these simple cooked chicken strips covered in all that bagel prepared with new broccoli as an afterthought.

The three-fixing plunging sauce adds simply a smidgen of sweetness and zest.

Fixings

3 tablespoons extra-virgin olive oil, isolated

4 teaspoons of all that bagel preparing, isolated

½ teaspoon ground pepper, isolated

1 12-ounce bundle of broccoli florets (around 6 cups)

1 pound chicken fingers

⅓ cup low-fat plain Greek yogurt

1 tablespoon Dijon mustard

2 teaspoons honey

Instructions

Place the rack in the upper third of the broiler. Preheat the oven to high. Line a large rimmed baking sheet with foil.

Consolidate 2 tablespoons oil, 2 teaspoons bagel preparation, and ¼ teaspoon pepper in a huge bowl. Add broccoli; mix to cover, then spread equally on one portion of the pre-arranged baking sheet.

Join the leftover 1 tablespoon oil, 2 teaspoons bagel preparation, and 1 / 4 teaspoon pepper in the bowl. Add chicken and mix to cover. Orchestrate on the unfilled side of the baking sheet. Sear, turning the dish once, until the chicken is cooked through and the broccoli is delicate and caramelized, around 8 minutes.

In the meantime, join yogurt, mustard, and honey in a little bowl. Serve the pepper sauce with the broccoli and chicken.

6.   Simmered   Pistachio-Crusted Salmon with Broccoli

This simple one-skillet simmered salmon with broccoli is speedy enough for weeknight suppers however exquisite enough for the organization. The lemony pistachio hull would likewise be exquisite on different sorts of fish or on chicken bosoms.

Fixings

8 cups broccoli florets with 2-inch stalks appended

Fixing

2 cloves garlic, cut

3 tablespoons extra-virgin olive oil, partitioned

¾ teaspoon salt, partitioned

½ teaspoon ground pepper, partitioned

½ cup salted pistachios, coarsely cleaved

2 tablespoons cleaved new chives

Zing of 1 medium lemon, in addition to wedges for serving

4 teaspoons mayonnaise

1 ¼ pounds salmon filet, cut into 4 segments

Instructions

Preheat broiler to 425 degrees F. Cover an enormous rimmed baking sheet with a cooking shower.

Consolidate broccoli, garlic, 2 tablespoons oil, 1/2 teaspoon salt, and 1/4 teaspoon pepper on the pre-arranged baking sheet. Broil for 5 minutes.

In the meantime, consolidate pistachios, chives, lemon zing, the leftover 1 tablespoon oil, and 1/4 teaspoon each salt and pepper in a little bowl. Spread 1 teaspoon of mayonnaise over every salmon part and top with the pistachio blend.

Move the broccoli aside from the baking sheet and put the salmon on the vacant side. Cook until the salmon is murky in the middle and the broccoli is simply delicate, 8 to 15 minutes more, contingent upon thickness. Present with lemon wedges, whenever wanted.

7. Sheet-Container Teriyaki Tofu with Carrots and Broccoli

With only one sheet container and 35 minutes, you can get a delightful veggie lover supper on the table. The carrots get an early advantage in the broiler to guarantee they are cooked through, while a sprinkle of teriyaki sauce toward the end integrates everything. Present with earthy colored rice, whenever wanted.

Fixings

1 pound carrots, cut on the predisposition 1/2-inch thick

2 tablespoons extra-virgin olive oil, partitioned

¾ teaspoon salt, separated

¾ teaspoon ground pepper, separated

2 cups broccoli florets

2 cups cut red chime pepper

1 (16-ounce) bundle of tofu, depleted, squeezed, and cubed (1/2-to 3/4-inch)

1 teaspoon curry powder

3 tablespoons low-sodium teriyaki sauce

Instructions

Position the rack in the lower third of the stove; preheat to 425°F.

Throw carrots with 1 tablespoon of oil and 1/4 teaspoon each salt and pepper in an enormous bowl. Spread uniformly on an enormous rimmed baking sheet. Broil for 15 minutes.

Throw broccoli and ringer pepper with the leftover 1 tablespoon oil and 1/4 teaspoon each salt and pepper in the bowl. Mix into the carrots on the baking sheet.

Sprinkle tofu with curry powder and the excess 1/4 teaspoon each salt and pepper. Orchestrate on top of the vegetables. Cook until the tofu is beginning to brown and the vegetables are delicate, 10 to 15 minutes.

Move the tofu and vegetables to a serving platter; shower with teriyaki sauce.

8. Cooked Salmon with Smoky Chickpeas and Greens

Fixings

2 tablespoons extra-virgin olive oil, partitioned

1 tablespoon smoked paprika

½ teaspoon salt, partitioned, in addition to a squeeze

1 (15 ounces) can no-salt-added chickpeas, flushed

⅓ cup buttermilk

¼ cup mayonnaise

¼ cup cleaved new chives as well as dill, in addition to something else for decorating

½ teaspoon ground pepper, partitioned

¼ teaspoon garlic powder

10 cups cleaved kale

¼ cup water

1 ¼ pounds wild salmon, cut into 4 segments

Instructions

Position racks in the upper third and center of the broiler; preheat to 425 degrees F.

Consolidate 1 tablespoon oil, paprika, and 1/4 teaspoon salt in a medium bowl. Completely wipe the chickpeas off, then throw with the paprika combination. Spread on a rimmed baking sheet. Prepare the chickpeas on the upper rack, blending two times, for 30 minutes.

In the meantime, puree buttermilk, mayonnaise, spices, 1/4 teaspoon pepper, and garlic powder in a blender until smooth. Put away.

Heat the excess 1 tablespoon oil in an enormous skillet over medium intensity. Add kale and cook, mixing infrequently, for 2 minutes. Add water and keep cooking until the kale is delicate, around 5 minutes more. Eliminate from intensity and mix when necessary with salt.

Eliminate the chickpeas from the broiler and push them aside from the dish. Put salmon on the opposite side and season with the excess 1/4 teaspoon each salt and pepper. Prepare until the salmon is simply cooked through, 5 to 8 minutes.

Shower the held dressing on the salmon, decorate with additional spices, whenever wanted, and present with the kale and chickpeas.

9. Sheet-Container Lemon-Pepper Chicken with Broccoli and Tomatoes

This sheet-container lemon-pepper chicken with broccoli and tomatoes offers a mix of nutrient-rich vegetables, a solid portion of fiber, and lean protein to fill your plate. Lemon pepper season the dish, adding brilliance and zest.

How We Made This Diabetes-appropriate

1. The bones and skin from bone-in, skin-on chicken bosom trap a portion of the dampness inside the meat, keeping it from drying out

while it's cooking. Chicken bosom is a normally lean protein, with the vast majority of the fat tracked down in the skin. To scale back soaked fat, you can eliminate the skin after it's finished cooking.

2. Without salt flavoring is a low-sodium food that permits you to add salt (and saltier fixings like feta cheddar) in different places so the flavor is spread equitably all through the dish. An excess of sodium admission is related to hypertension and an expanded gamble of cardiovascular sickness.

Tips from the Test Kitchen

How might I at any point make this veggie lover?
You can add extra-firm tofu in place of the chicken, or attempt a container of no-salt-added chickpeas, which will get decent and crunchy as they cook.

What can I at any point use for all things being equal? I can't find any without salt lemon-pepper preparation.
You can consolidate the zing of 1 lemon (around 1 tablespoon) and 1 teaspoon pepper.

What would it be advisable for me to present with this?
This dish is perfect all alone yet, in addition, can be presented with earthy colored rice or pureed potatoes, or on top of entire grain pasta.

What different vegetables can I at any point use rather than broccoli and cherry tomatoes?
You can utilize green beans, asparagus, cauliflower, zucchini, or summer squash. Delicate veggies like green beans and asparagus

will require less time on the stove, so add them later on to abstain from overcooking.

Fixings

8 cups broccoli florets

1 16 ounces cherry tomatoes

3 tablespoons extra-virgin olive oil, partitioned

½ teaspoon genuine salt, separated

¼ teaspoon ground pepper

1 ½ pounds bone-in, skin-on chicken bosomsx

2 teaspoons without salt lemon pepper preparing

⅓ cup disintegrated feta cheddar

Instructions

Preheat the stove to 425°F.

Throw broccoli and tomatoes in an enormous bowl with 2 tablespoons of oil, 1/4 teaspoon salt and pepper.

Cut chicken bosoms into 4 equivalent parts. Brush the chicken with the leftover 1 tablespoon oil and sprinkle with lemon pepper preparation and the excess 1/4 teaspoon salt. Put the chicken on one portion of a rimmed baking sheet. Broil for 10 minutes. Eliminate from stove; cautiously add the broccoli and tomatoes to the opposite side of the dish.

Keep boiling, blending the vegetables once part of the way through, until a moment read the thermometer embedded in the thickest piece of a bosom without contacting bone registers 165°F, and the vegetables are delicate, 15 to 18 minutes more. Sprinkle feta over the vegetables on the skillet; mix to permit the feta to soften somewhat. Serve the chicken and vegetables finished off with the skillet drippings.

10. Sheet-Skillet Sesame Chicken and Broccoli with Scallion-Ginger Sauce

Fixings

8 cups broccoli florets with 2-inch stalks joined

2 tablespoons sesame oil, separated

1 teaspoon salt, separated

½ teaspoon ground pepper, separated

2 pounds bone-in chicken thighs, managed

2 tablespoons avocado oil

3 tablespoons minced scallion

2 teaspoons minced new ginger

1 teaspoon rice vinegar

2 teaspoons toasted sesame seeds

Instructions

Place a huge rimmed baking sheet on the stove. Preheat the stove to 425 degrees F.

Consolidate broccoli, 1 tablespoon of sesame oil, and 1/4 teaspoon each salt and pepper in an enormous bowl. Throw chicken with the leftover 1 tablespoon of sesame oil and 1/4 teaspoon each salt and pepper in another bowl.

Place the chicken skin-side-down in a solitary layer on one side of the preheated skillet. Broil for 15 minutes. Turn the chicken over and add the broccoli to the opposite side of the skillet. Keep cooking, turning the broccoli part of the way through, until the chicken is simply cooked through and the broccoli is delicate, 20 to 25 minutes more.

In the meantime, heat a little skillet over medium-high intensity until practically smoking. Add avocado oil, scallion, ginger, vinegar, and the leftover 1/2 teaspoon salt; cook, mixing, for 15 seconds. Eliminate from heat.

Serve the chicken and broccoli showered with the scallion-ginger sauce and sprinkled with sesame seeds.

11. Sheet-Dish Lemon-Garlic Salmon with Delicata and Kale

Fixings

1 pound delicata squash, split longwise, cultivated, and cut (1/2-inch)

2 tablespoons extra-virgin olive oil, partitioned

¾ teaspoon salt, partitioned

¾ teaspoon ground pepper, partitioned

6 cups coarsely cleaved stemmed kale

1 ¼ pounds cleaned salmon, cut into 4 segments

½ teaspoon dried dill

½ teaspoon garlic powder

3 tablespoons lemon juice

Instructions

Position rack in the lower third of broiler; preheat to 425°F.

Throw squash with 1 tablespoon oil and 1/4 teaspoon each salt and pepper in a huge bowl. Spread uniformly on an enormous rimmed baking sheet. Broil for 15 minutes.

Throw kale with the leftover 1 tablespoon oil and 1/4 teaspoon each salt and pepper in the bowl. Mix into the squash on the baking sheet.

Sprinkle salmon with dill, garlic powder, and the excess 1/4 teaspoon each salt and pepper. Put the salmon on top of the vegetables. Broil until the salmon is cooked through and chips effectively and the vegetables are delicate, 10 to 15 minutes.

Move the salmon and vegetables to a serving platter; sprinkle with lemon juice.

12. Sheet-Container Bean stew Lime Salmon with Potatoes and Peppers

Fixings
1 pound Yukon Gold potatoes, cut into 3/4-inch pieces
2 tablespoons extra-virgin olive oil, partitioned
¾ teaspoon salt, partitioned
¼ teaspoon ground pepper
2 teaspoons bean stew powder
1 teaspoon ground cumin
½ teaspoon garlic powder
1 lime, zested and quartered
2 medium ringer peppers, any tone, cut
1 ¼ pounds focus cut salmon filet, cleaned, whenever wanted and cut into 4 bits

Instructions

Preheat the broiler to 425 degrees F. Cover a huge rimmed baking sheet with a cooking splash.

Throw potatoes, 1 tablespoon oil, 1/4 teaspoon salt, and pepper together in a medium bowl. Move to the pre-arranged dish and meal for 15 minutes.

In the meantime, join bean stew powder, cumin, garlic powder, lime zing, and the leftover 1/2 teaspoon salt in a little bowl. Place chime peppers in the medium bowl and add the excess 1 tablespoon oil and 1/2 tablespoon of the flavor blend; throw well to cover. Cover the salmon with the excess zest blend.

After 15 minutes, eliminate the container from the stove. Add the peppers and mix to join. Broil for 5 minutes. Eliminate from the stove; move a portion of the vegetables over and add the salmon to the container. Broil until the salmon is simply cooked through, 6 to 8 minutes. Present with lime wedges.

13. Ginger-Tahini Stove Heated Salmon and Vegetables

Fixings

1 huge yam, cubed (around 12 oz.)

1 pound of white button or cremini mushrooms, cut into 1-inch pieces (6 cups)

2 tablespoons olive oil, separated

½ teaspoon salt, separated

1 pound green beans, managed

2 tablespoons decreased sodium soy sauce

3 tablespoon of tahini

2 tablespoon of honey

1 ½ teaspoons finely ground new ginger

1 ¼ pounds salmon, ideally wild-got, cut into 4 bits

2 teaspoons rice vinegar

2 tablespoons slashed new chives (Discretionary)

Instructions

Place an enormous rimmed baking sheet in the broiler. Position one rack on the stove and one more around 6 creeps from the grill. Preheat to 425 degrees F.

Consolidate yam, mushrooms, 1 Tbsp. oil, and 1/4 tsp. salt in an enormous bowl; throw to cover.

Eliminate the baking sheet from the broiler. Spread the vegetable blend in an even layer on the skillet; broil, blending once until the yams are beginning to brown, around 20 minutes.
In the interim, throw green beans with the leftover 1 Tbsp. oil and 1/4 tsp. salt.
Add soy sauce, tahini, honey, and ginger in a little bowl.

Eliminate the skillet from the stove. Place the mushrooms and yams aside and put the green beans on the opposite side. Place salmon in the center, nestling it on top of the vegetables, if fundamental. Spread a portion of the tahini sauce on top of the salmon. Cook until the salmon pieces, 8 to 10 minutes more. Go oven to high; move the skillet to the top rack and sear until the salmon is coated, around 3 minutes.

Mix vinegar into the leftover tahini sauce and shower it over the salmon and vegetables. Embellish with chives, whenever wanted, and serve.

Tips

To make ahead: Get ready tahini sauce (Stage 4) as long as 1 day ahead; cover and refrigerate.

14. Sheet-Dish Shrimp and Beets

Fixings

1 pound little beets, stripped and cut into 1/2-inch pieces

2 tablespoons extra-virgin olive oil, separated

¾ teaspoon salt, separated

¾ teaspoon ground pepper, separated

6 cups packed kale

1 ¼ pounds extra-huge crude shrimp (16-20 count), stripped and deveined

½ teaspoon dry mustard

½ teaspoon dried tarragon

3 tablespoons unsalted sunflower seeds, toasted

Instructions

Preheat the stove to 425 degrees F.

Throw beets with 1 tablespoon of oil and 1/4 teaspoon each salt and pepper in a huge bowl. Spread uniformly on a rimmed baking sheet. Broil for 15 minutes.

Throw kale with the excess 1 tablespoon oil and 1/4 teaspoon each salt and pepper in the bowl. Mix into the beets on the baking sheet.

Sprinkle shrimp with mustard, tarragon, and the leftover 1/4 teaspoon each salt and pepper. Put on top of the vegetables. Broil until the shrimp are cooked and the vegetables are delicate, 10 to 15 minutes more.

Move the shrimp to a serving platter. Mix sunflower seeds into the vegetables and present with the shrimp.

15. Mediterranean Chicken and Vegetable Bake

Ingredients
4 boneless, skinless chicken bosoms
2 cups cherry tomatoes
1 red ringer pepper, cut
1 yellow ringer pepper, cut
1 red onion, cut
2 cloves garlic, minced
2 tablespoons olive oil
1 teaspoon dried oregano
Salt and pepper to taste

Instructions

Preheat your stove to 400°F (200°C).

In a huge bowl, consolidate chicken, vegetables, garlic, olive oil, oregano, salt, and pepper.

Spread the blend on a sheet dish and prepare for 25-30 minutes, or until the chicken is cooked through.

16. Mediterranean Salmon and Asparagus

Ingredients

4 salmon filets

1 bundle of asparagus, managed

1 lemon, cut

2 cloves garlic, minced

2 tablespoons olive oil

1 teaspoon dried thyme

Salt and pepper to taste

Instruction

Preheat your broiler to 400°F (200°C).

In a bowl, blend olive oil, garlic, thyme, salt, and pepper.

Put salmon filets and asparagus on a sheet dish, shower with the olive oil combination, and top with lemon cuts.

Heat for 12-15 minutes or until salmon drops without any problem.

17. Mediterranean Broiled Veggie Platter

Ingredients

2 zucchinis, cut

2 red chime peppers, cut

1 red onion, cut

1 cup cherry tomatoes

1 can chickpeas, depleted and washed

3 tablespoons olive oil

2 teaspoons dried basil

 Salt and pepper to taste

Instructions

Preheat your stove to 425°F (220°C).

Throw every one of the vegetables and chickpeas with olive oil, basil, salt, and pepper.

Spread them equally on a sheet dish and meal for 25-30 minutes, or until the vegetables are delicate.

18. Mediterranean Shrimp and Quinoa

Ingredients

1 pound huge shrimp, stripped and deveined
1 cup quinoa, washed
2 cups chicken or vegetable stock
1 zucchini, diced
1 red chime pepper, diced
1 yellow chime pepper, diced
2 tablespoons olive oil
1 teaspoon dried rosemary
Salt and pepper to taste

Instructions

Preheat your stove to 400°F (200°C).

In a baking dish, consolidate quinoa, stock, vegetables, olive oil, rosemary, salt, and pepper. Put shrimp on top and cover with foil. Prepare for 20-25 minutes until the shrimp is pink and cooked through.

19. Mediterranean Tofu and Veggie Bake

Ingredients

1 block of extra-firm tofu, cubed
1 cup cherry tomatoes
1 red onion, cut
1 red ringer pepper, cut
1 yellow ringer pepper, cut
2 cloves garlic, minced

2 tablespoons olive oil

1 teaspoon dried thyme

Salt and pepper to taste

Instructions

Preheat your broiler to 400°F (200°C).

In a bowl, throw tofu, vegetables, garlic, olive oil, thyme, salt, and pepper.

Spread the combination on a sheet skillet and heat for 20-25 minutes or until tofu is fresh.

20. Mediterranean Sheep and Potatoes

Ingredients

1 pound sheep slashes

4 potatoes, cut into lumps

1 red onion, cut

4 cloves garlic, minced

2 tablespoons olive oil

1 teaspoon dried rosemary

Salt and pepper to taste

Instructions

Preheat your broiler to 425°F (220°C).

In a bowl, consolidate sheep, potatoes, onion, garlic, olive oil, rosemary, salt, and pepper.

Spread the combination on a sheet dish and meal for 30-35 minutes, or until the sheep is cooked to your ideal doneness.

21. Mediterranean Cooked Cod and Veggies

Ingredients

4 cod filets

1 cup cherry tomatoes

1 zucchini, cut

1 yellow squash, cut

1 red onion, cut

2 tablespoons olive oil

1 teaspoon dried basil

Salt and pepper to taste

Instructions

Preheat your broiler to 400°F (200°C).

In a bowl, combine cod, vegetables, olive oil, basil, salt, and pepper.

Put the blend on a sheet dish and prepare for 15-20 minutes or until the cod chips are without any problem.

CONCLUSION

These sheet-skillet meals are delightful as well as in accordance with the Mediterranean eating routine, which is rich in organic products, vegetables, lean proteins, and sound fats known to assist with diminishing aggravation. Enjoy!

9 7 9 8 8 6 2 4 2 7 8 2 0